Sirtfood Diet Guide

Shed Weight, Burn fat and Energize your Body by Activating your "Skinny" Gene

Jane Harris

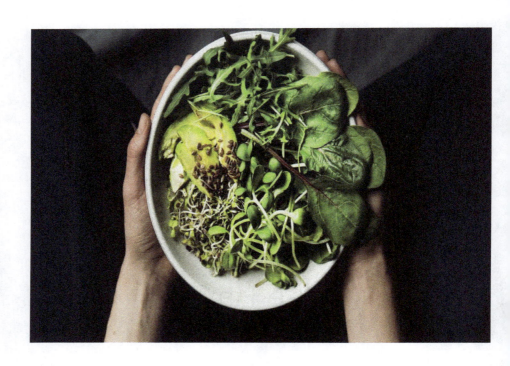

© **Copyright 2021 Jane Harris- All rights reserved.**

The content contained within this book may not be reproduced, duplicated or transmitted without direct written permission from the author or the publisher.

Under no circumstances will any blame or legal responsibility be held against the publisher, or author, for any damages, reparation, or monetary loss due to the information contained within this book. Either directly or indirectly.

Legal Notice:

This book is copyright protected. This book is only for personal use. You cannot amend, distribute, sell, use, quote or paraphrase any part, or the content within this book, without the consent of the author or publisher.

Disclaimer Notice:

Please note the information contained within this document is for educational and entertainment purposes only. All effort has been executed to present accurate, up to date, and reliable, complete information. No warranties of any kind are declared or implied. Readers acknowledge that the author is not engaging in the rendering of legal, financial, medical or professional advice. The content within this book has been derived from various sources. Please consult a licensed professional before attempting any techniques outlined in this book.

By reading this document, the reader agrees that under no circumstances is the author responsible for any losses, direct or indirect, which are incurred as a result of the use of information contained within this document, including, but not limited to, - errors, omissions, or inaccuracies.

Contents

WHAT IS THE SIRTFOOD DIET? 1

PHASES OF THE SIRTFOOD DIET 8

The Best 20 Sirtfoods 14

FAQ 25

SIRTFOOD FOR BUILDING 30

BENEFITS OF SIRTFOOD DIET 36

MAIN DISHES 46

Green Beans With Crispy Chickpeas 46

Sloppy Joe Scramble Stuffed Spuds 48

Baked Salmon Salad With Creamy Mint Dressing 51

Fragrant Asian Hot Pot 53

Tofu Scramble With Mushrooms 55

Prawn Arrabbiata 57

Turmeric Baked Salmon 59

Baked Potatoes With Spicy Chickpea Stew 61

Kale And Red Onion Dhal With Buckwheat 63

Kale, Edamame And Tofu Curry 66

Lemon Chicken With Spinach, Red Onion, And Salsa 68

Smoked Salmon Omelet 70

Broccoli And Pasta 71

Artichokes and Kale with Walnuts 73

Tuna And Tomatoes 77

Salmon & Kale Omelet 80

Moroccan Spiced Eggs 82

Chili Sweetcorn And Wild Garlic Fritters 86

Roast Mackerel And Simple Veggies 88
Baked Root Veg With Chili 90
Autumn Stuffed Enchiladas 93
Creamy Vegetable Casserole 96
Vegan Mac And Cheese 99
Butternut Squash Alfredo 101
Cajun Turkey Rice 104
Tomato & Goat's Cheese Pizza 106

WHAT IS THE SIRTFOOD DIET?

Sirtuins are a group of proteins that manage cell wellbeing. Sirtuins assume a key job in controlling cell homeostasis.

In the cells, numerous pieces are taking a shot at different undertakings with an extreme objective, as well: remain sound and capacity proficiently for whatever length of time that conceivable. Similarly, as needs in the organization change, because of different inside and outer variables, so do needs in the cells. Somebody needs to run the workplace, directing what completes when, who will do it and when to switch course.

NAD+ is essential to cell digestion and many other organic procedures. If sirtuins are an organization's CEO, at that point, NAD+ is the cash that pays the pay of the CEO and workers, all while keeping the lights on and the workplace space lease paid. An organization, and the body, can't work without it.

Protein may seem like dietary protein — what's found in beans and meats and well, protein shakes — yet for this situation we're discussing atoms called proteins, which work all through the body's phones in various capacities.

Consider proteins the divisions at an organization, everyone concentrating without anyone else explicit capacity while planning with different offices.

Acetyl groups control explicit responses. They're physical labels on proteins that different proteins perceive will respond with them. If proteins are the branches of the cell and DNA are the CEO, the acetyl groups are the accessibility status of every division head. For instance, if a protein is accessible, at that point the sirtuins can work with it to get something going; similarly, as the CEO can work with an accessible division head to get something going.

Sirtuins work with acetyl groups by doing what's called deacetylation. One way that sirtuins work is by evacuating acetyl gatherings deacetylation organic proteins, for example, histones. The histone is an enormous cumbersome protein that the DNA folds itself over. This loosened up chromatin implies the DNA is being translated, a fundamental procedure.

We've just thought about sirtuins for around 20 years, and their essential capacity was found during the 1990s. From that point forward, specialists have rushed to examine them, recognizing their significance while likewise bringing up issues about what else we can find out about them.

In 1991, Elysium fellow benefactor and MIT scientist Leonard Guarantee, along with graduate understudies Nick Austria and Brian Kennedy, directed tests to all the more likely see how yeast matured. By some coincidence, Austria attempted to develop societies of different yeast strains from tests he had put away in his ice chest for quite a long time, which made an unpleasant situation for the strains.

This is the place acetyl groups become possibly the most important factor. It was their first idea that SIR2 may be a deacetylation protein — which means it expelled those acetyl gatherings — from different atoms, however, nobody knew whether this was valid since all endeavors to show this movement in a test tube demonstrated negative.

In Guarantee's very own words: "Without NAD+, SIR2 sirts idle. That was the basic finding on the circular segment of sirtuins science."

Ecological factors significantly influence the destiny of living beings and sustenance is one of the most persuasive variables. These days life span is a significant objective of medicinal science and has consistently been a fabrication for the individual since antiquated occasions. Specifically, endeavors are planned for accomplishing effective maturing, to be a long life without genuine ailments, with a decent degree of physical and mental autonomy and satisfactory social connections.

Gathering information unmistakably exhibits that it is conceivable to impact the indications of maturing. Without a doubt, wholesome mediations can advance wellbeing and life span. A tribute must be given to Ansel Keys, who was the first to give strong logical proof about the job of sustenance in the wellbeing/sickness balance at the populace level, explicitly in connection to cardiovascular illness, still the main source of death overall. It is commonly valued that the sort of diet can significantly impact the quality and amount of life and the Mediterranean eating regimen is paradigmatic of an advantageous

dietary example. The developing cognizance of the useful impacts of a particular dietary example on wellbeing and life span in the second half of the remaining century produced a ground-breaking push toward structuring eating fewer carbs that could diminish the danger of constant maladies, subsequently bringing about solid maturing. Subsequently, during the 1990s the Dietary Approaches to Stop Hypertension Dash diet was contrived to assess whether it was conceivable to treat hypertension not pharmacologically.

To be sure, the DASH diet was very like the Mediterranean Diet, being wealthy in foods grown from the ground, entire grains, and strands, while poor in creature soaked fats and cholesterol. The awesome news leaving the investigation was that not exclusively did the DASH diet lower circulatory strain, however, it additionally diminished the danger of cardiovascular infection, type 2 diabetes, a few sorts of malignant growth, and other maturing related maladies. To additionally improve the medical advantages of plant nourishment rich, creature fat-terrible eating routines, especially in people with hypercholesterolemia, the Portfolio Diet was planned.

This eating regimen, other than being to a great extent veggielover, with just limited quantities of soaked fats, prescribes likewise a high admission of utilitarian nourishments, including thick filaments, plant stools, soy proteins, and almonds. Curiously, members on the Portfolio Diet displayed a decrease of coronary illness chance related to lower plasma cholesterol in contrast with members on a sound, for the most part, vegan diet.

Additionally, the measure of ingested nourishment has been pulling in lightof a legitimate concern for mainstream researchers as a potential modifier of the harmony among wellbeing and infection in a wide range of living species.

Specifically, calorie limitation CR has been exhibited to be a rising healthful intercession that animates the counter maturing instruments in the body.

In this way, the eating routine of the individuals living on the Japanese island of Okinawa has been widely broken down because these islanders are notable for their life span and expanded wellbeing range, bringing about the best recurrence of centenarians on the planet. Interestingly, the customary Okinawan diet came about to be fundamentally the same as the Mediterranean Diet and the DASH diet regarding nourishment types.

Be that as it may, the vitality admission of Okinawans, at the hour of the underlying logical perceptions, was about 20% lower than the normal vitality admission of the Japanese, along these lines deciding an average state of CR.

Singer Adele has confirmed that she has lost 30 kilos in just one year. The secret? It's all thanks to the Sirtfood Diet. It was revealed by the singer herself through international media, such as the Daily Mail and the New York Post.

The Sirtfood Diet is not the classic fasting diet: Adele is the living proof of this, given the splendid shape in which was at her appointments with her fans.

It is, in fact, a diet that leaves room for both cheese and red wine as well as chocolate, in the right proportions, and of course under the supervision of a specialist doctor, who knows how to evaluate your health and recommend the most suitable diet to lose weight safely.

Many were the media that underlined the substantial weight loss of the singer Adele who admitted how the decision to lose weight did not depend on the acceptance of her as much as the difficulty of using her voice to the fullest.

Adele praised the Sirtfood Diet, which made her lose 30 kilos without much

effort although, in reality, she admitted via Instagram that she had never struggled as much in physical activity as when preparing for her tour. She also said that the beauty of Sirtfoods is that many of them are already on our table every day. They are accessible and can be easily integrated into our diet.

PHASES OF THE SIRTFOOD DIET

The diet is mainly divided into two phases: the first lasts one week and the other lasts 14 days.

Phase 1 (The Most Effective): Three Kilos in Seven Days

It is the "supersonic" phase: the calorie restriction is combined with a diet rich in Sirt foods. The novelty compared to other diets is that it fattens and fattens the muscles. Two different moments. Days 1-3 are the most intense, and during this time you can consume a maximum of one thousand calories per day. You must consume 3 Sirt green juices and a solid meal.

On days 4-7 assigned the intake of one thousand five hundred calories daily.

You have to take two green Sirt juices and two solid meals. Phase 1 is the most intense, in which the best results are seen and which allows you to lose up to 3.5 kilos.

The maximum of calories consumed during the first 3 days is 1000, while from the fourth to the seventh one reaches 1500 calories per day.

The menu to follow includes a "fixed" part, the one relating to green juice created by nutritionists that helps to moderate the appetite of the brain, and one that varies daily.

The green juice recipe is simple and includes all-natural products: 75 g of curly kale, 30 g of arugula and 5 g of parsley must be centrifuged, together with 150 g of green celery with the leaves and 1/2 green apple, grated.

Everything must be completed with half a squeezed lemon and half a teaspoon of Matcha tea.

Here is more in detail the program of the first week:

Monday - Wednesday: 3 Sirt green juices to be taken on waking up, midmorning and mid-afternoon; 1 solid meal of animal or vegan protein (for example, turkey escalope or buckwheat noodles with tofu) accompanied by vegetables, always ending with 15-20 g of 85% dark chocolate.

Thursday - Sunday: 2 Sirt green juices and 2 solid meals, remembering to always vary the main course chosen, from salmon fillet to vegetable tabbouleh to buckwheat spaghetti with celery and kale.

Phase 2 (Maintenance), For 14 Days

Every day, for 14 days, you will eat three balanced meals, chock full of Sirt foods, drink a Sirt green juice, and consume 1-2 Sirt snacks. Green juice should be taken in the morning as soon as you wake up or at least 30 minutes before breakfast, or mid-morning. The evening meal must be eaten by 7 pm.

Phase 2 is the maintenance phase. During this period the goal is the consolidation of the weight loss, although the possibility of losing weight is not excluded. To do all this, just feed on the exceptional foods rich in sirtuins.

It lasts 14 days, it is less restrictive than the first and provides for sirt foods at will: 3 solid meals plus two juices. The important thing is that they are balanced.

The positive aspects of this diet are:

One is the fact that the calorie limit is indicative and not a goal to be achieved. Another advantage is that the dishes on offer are very satisfying.

This way you won't have the hunger attacks typical of other diets. The caloric restriction of the diet even in the most intensive phase is not drastic and Sirt foods have a satiating effect, which prevents us from getting hungry at meals

And then?

As already explained in the introduction, the Sirtfood diet cannot (and must not) continue indefinitely and for a very long time. Rather, it must be done in cycles, once, two, or three times a year. However, the sirt "lifestyle" can continue even after completing the phase.

Sirt foods can be eaten all year round, continuing to speed up the metabolism.

However, this should not be combined with a very strong calorie restriction, but only avoid eating unhealthy foods, such as fried, sweet, or unsaturated fats. Your persistence will make the difference between success and failure, remember: this is not a shot, but a marathon!

Sirt cycles are simply a boost, a powerful weapon in your arsenal that you can use twice a year (depending on your body of course), but you can have a healthy lifestyle all year round, perhaps combined with regular physical exercise.

Phase 3 (Make the Sirt Food Diet For Life)

For 1 week, the participants followed the diet and exercised daily. At the end of the week, participants lost an average of 7 pounds (3.2 kg) and maintained or even gained muscle mass.

Yet, these results are hardly surprising. Restricting your calorie intake to 1,000 calories and exercising at the same time will nearly always cause weight loss.

Regardless, this kind of quick weight loss is neither genuine nor long-lasting, and this study did not follow participants after the first week to see if they gained any of the weight back, which is typically the case.

When your body is energy-deprived, it uses up its emergency energy stores, or glycogen, in addition to burning fat and muscle.

Each molecule of glycogen requires 3–4 molecules of water to be stored.

When your body uses up glycogen, it gets rid of this water as well. It's known as "water weight."

In the first week of extreme calorie restriction, only about one-third of the weight loss comes from fat, while the other two-thirds come from water, muscle, and glycogen. As soon as your calorie intake increases, your body replenishes its glycogen stores, and the weight comes right back.

Unfortunately, this type of calorie restriction can also cause your body to lower its metabolic rate, causing you to need even fewer calories per day for energy than before.

This diet may likely help you lose a few pounds in the beginning, but it'll likely come back as soon as the diet is over. As far as preventing disease, 3 weeks is probably not long enough to have any measurable long-term impact.

On the other hand, adding Sirtfoods to your regular diet over the long term may very well be a good idea. But in that case, you might as well skip the diet and start doing that now.

The Best 20 Sirtfoods
Arugula

This green salad leaf (also known as rucola) is very common in the Mediterranean diet. It is not too popular in the US food culture, and it is considered an absolute arrogance to have it on your plate. However, we are not talking about a leaf covered in gold or silver; we are talking about a green salad leaf with a peppery taste that can be used for digestive and diuretic purposes. During the time of ancient Rome and in the middle Ages, this leaf was known to have aphrodisiac properties.

However, there is a lot more to this miracle leaf. It has nutrients like quercetin and kaempferol capable of activating sirtuins. This combination is said to have very positive effects on the skin as it can moisturize and improve collagen synthesis. So why not have this leaf in your salad and add some extra olive oil on it, making it a powerful Sirtfood duo? As you can see, it has many positive effects on your body.

Buckwheat

This is one of the best sources for rutin, a sirtuin-activator nutrient. However, this crop is also amazing for ecological and sustainable farming, as it can improve the quality of the soil and prevent weed growth. However, probably the most interesting part about buckwheat is that it is a fruit seed, kind of like rhubarb, so it is not a grain at all. It is not a coincidence at all that buckwheat has more protein than any grain known to man, so it fits perfectly in your Sirtfood diet. For every person trying to avoid gluten, this can be the ideal food. It is the ideal alternative for grains.

Capers

Some of you may not be too familiar with capers. If you have not had the chance to taste them, you should. They are those dark-green salty things you can see sometimes on top of a pizza.

Unfortunately, capers are not very used in a standard diet (it is very overlooked and underrated), but those who never had the chance to try capers do not know what they are missing. We are talking about the flower buds of the caper bush, a plant growing abundantly in the Mediterranean region. It is usually handpicked and preserved, and it has some interesting antidiabetic, anti-inflammatory, antimicrobial, antiviral, and immunomodulatory properties. Moreover, it has been used in medicine all around the Mediterranean area.

Celery

This is a plant used for thousands of years, as in ancient Egypt, people were already aware of it and its properties. Back then, it was considered a medicinal plant that can be used for detoxing, cleansing and preventing diseases. Therefore, celery consumption is very good for your gut, kidney, and liver. When it was growing wildly in ancient times, it had a strong bitter flavor. However, ever since its domestication in the 17th century, celery has become a bit sweeter, and now it can be used in salads.

Chilies

This veggie should be in your diet whether you like eating spicy food or not.

It contains capsaicin, and this substance makes us savor it even more.

Consuming chilies is great for activating sirtuins and it speeds up your metabolism. In fact, the spicier the chili is, the more powerful it is when it comes to activating sirtuins. You probably heard that people eating spicy food three or four times per week have a 14 percent lower death rate compared to people who eat them less than once a week. Now, this does not mean that you have to go for the hottest chilies you can find, especially if you are not a spicy food enthusiast. Take it easy at the beginning.

Cocoa

The Aztecs and Mayans considered Cocoa sacred, and it was a food type reserved only for the warriors or the elite. It was often used as a currency, as people were aware of its value.

Although back then it was mostly used as a drink, you do not have to dilute it with milk or water to reap the full benefits of it. The best way to consume cocoa is by eating dark chocolate (with at least 85 percent solid cocoa).

However, this also depends on how the chocolate is made, as this product is usually treated with an alkalizing agent, which is known to lower the acidity of the chocolate and give a darker color. This substance is also known to reduce the sirtuin-activating flavanols.

Coffee

This is a drink enjoyed by most adults out there, and it is considered indispensable by most of them. We even believe that we can function without a cup of coffee to start within the morning. Obviously, that is not true, but we can honestly believe that coffee significantly improves our productivity and our daily activities.

Caffeine acid is a nutrient known to activate sirtuins, so there is more to drinking coffee than a popular and very pleasant social activity.

Extra Virgin Olive Oil

This oil is perhaps the healthiest form of fats you can think of, and it is not missing from any salad in the Mediterranean diet. The health benefits of consuming this oil are countless. It prevents and fights against diabetes, different types of cancer, osteoporosis, and many more. Besides, EVO oil can be associated with increased longevity, as it also has anti-aging effects. You can easily find this type of oil in most supermarkets, so you do not have any excuse to exclude it from your Sirtfood diet. This oil has the right nutrients to activate the sirtuin gene in your body.

Garlic

I do not know about you people, but I am simply in love with garlic. I am sure I am not the only one. Forget about the smell it leaves behind. Enjoy the great taste it offers. I would have garlic with any meal. Of course, this may not fit with our busy lifestyle, as it is not recommended to have it before a meeting, but you can enjoy it for dinner or at home. However, there is more to the consumption of garlic. As you probably know, it has an antifungal and antibiotic effect and has been successfully used to treat stomach ulcers. Also, it can be used to remove waste products from your body.

Green Tea

In some cultures, drinking tea is as popular as drinking coffee, but what if you find the tea assortment that works best for you. You can indeed have tea from various medicinal plants, and they all have positive effects on your health. However, most of these plants are focused on preventing or fighting a specific disease. Have you ever thought about drinking tea for your well-being or to feel great? Well, this is what green tea is for. First appeared in Asia, green tea has become very popular in Western culture. It has plenty of antioxidants. It can be used for detox, and it speeds up your metabolism.

Kale

You can never go wrong with some leafy greens, and this is applicable for kale as well. Perhaps not many of you have tried it before, but it is totally worth it. Over the last few years, kale has gained a lot of popularity and appreciation from both nutritionists and consumers, and they have all the reasons to like and appreciate it.

Medjool Dates

If you have the chance to go to any country in the Middle East or the Arabian Peninsula, you will find that dates are a very common snack. Dehydrated, covered in chocolate, or a fresher form, dates are perhaps the most common snack you can find over there.

Parsley

The parsley leaves are extremely frequent in recipes, so it is not missing from the Sirtfood diet. You can chop them and toss them in your meal or use a sprig for decorative purposes. But parsley is not for decorating your plate, as you are not trying to impress a jury of famous chefs. This is an underrated plant.

Red Endive

This vegetable is one of the latest discoveries in the world of plants. How come? It was discovered by accident in 1830 when a Belgian farmer who stored chicory roots in his cellar, forgot about them and discovered them with white leaves that happened to be crunchy, tender, and delicious.

Red Onions

If you are only eating onions as O-rings with your burger, then you had better rethink the way you consume this incredible vegetable. This type of onion has a sweeter taste (compared to yellow onion). It has plenty of antioxidants, and it is known to fight against inflammation, heart diseases, and diabetes.

Red Wine

The Mediterranean diet encourages the consumption of red wine, and there are plenty of reasons why you should consider the moderate consumption of it. We are not going to talk about the effects it has on your blood, blood sugar level, and so on. Not even about how moderate consumption can decrease the death rates by heart disease. Alternatively, about how red wine can prevent common colds and cavities (yes, it can even improve your oral health). Red wines like Merlot, Cabernet Sauvignon, or Pinot Noir have an incredible concentration of polyphenol to activate your sirtuins.

Soy

There is a completely food-processing industry behind soy, as it is used to create food products for vegetarians. However, let us face it — drinking soymilk will not activate your sirtuins. Industrially processed food is not very recommended for your health, so it should be excluded from your Sirtfood diet. In natural form, soy contains formononetin and daidzein, two great sirtuin-activating nutrients.

Strawberries

Of all the fruits out there, strawberries are among the ones with the most health benefits. Yes, they are sweet, but they happen to have a very high concentration of fisetin, a nutrient that can activate sirtuins. What is very confusing is that strawberries are known to prevent heart diseases, diabetes, cancer, osteoporosis, and Alzheimer's disease. They are even associated with healthy aging. Although they are sweet, 3½ ounces of strawberries only contain a teaspoon of sugar.

Turmeric

You are probably familiar with the effects ginger has on your overall health, but you do not know what turmeric can do for you. This plant is related to ginger, and it is very appreciated throughout Asia for medical and culinary reasons. India is responsible for 80 percent of the whole turmeric on the planet, and some nutritionists refer to it as the "golden spice" or "India's gold." Why is that? Because it contains curcumin, a very rare sirtuinactivating nutrient.

Walnuts

As it happens, the walnut tree is the oldest food tree known to humans, as it was discovered around 7,000 BCE. Its original location was in ancient Persia (modern-day Iran), and now this tree is spread all around the world, as it can easily adapt to different climates of the globe. In the United States, walnuts are a success story. California is the biggest producer of walnuts in the United States, responsible for 99 percent of the US commercial supply and three-quarters of the walnut trade worldwide.

FAQ
Can Children Eat Sirtfoods?

There are powerful Sirtfoods, most of which are safe for children. Obviously, children should avoid wine, coffee, and other highly caffeinated foods, such as matcha. On the other hand, children can enjoy sirtuin-rich foods such as cabbage, eggplant, blueberries, and dates with their regular balanced diet.

Yet, while children can enjoy most sirtuin-rich foods, that is not the same as to say that they can practice the Sirt diet. This diet plan is not designed for children, and it does not fit the needs of their growing bodies. Practicing this diet plan could not only negatively affect them physically, but it could damage their mental health for years to come. Anyone can develop an eating disorder, but it is especially true for children.

If you want your child to eat well, ensure they eat a wide range of foods, as recommended by their doctor, and you can simply include an abundance of sirtuin-rich foods into what they are already eating. Leave the focus on eating healthfully and not losing weight. Even if your child's doctor does want them to lose weight, you don't need to make the child aware of this fact. You can help guide them along with a healthy lifestyle, teaching them how to eat well and stay active through sports and play, and the weight will come off naturally without placing an unneeded burden on their small shoulders.

For similar reasons, you can include Sirtfoods in a balanced diet while pregnant, but you should avoid practicing the Sirt diet when you are pregnant. It doesn't contain the nutrition requirements for either a pregnant woman or a growing baby. Save the diet for after you have delivered a healthy baby, and both you and your child will be healthy and happy.

Can I Exercise During Phase One?

If you use exercise during either phase one or two, you can increase weight loss and health benefits. While you shouldn't work at pushing the limits during phase one, you can continue your normal workout routine and physical activity. It is important to stay within your active comfort zone during this time, as physical exertion more than you are accustomed to will be especially difficult while you are restricting your calories. It will not only wear you out, but it can also make you dizzy, more prone to injury, and physically and mentally exhausted. This is a common symptom whenever a person pushes their limits while restricting calories, but it is something you should avoid.

If you are used to doing yoga and a spin class a few times a week, keep it up!

If you are used to running a few miles a day, have at it! Do what you andbyour body are comfortable with, and as your doctor advises, and you should be fine.

I'm Already Thin. Can I Still Follow the Diet?

Whether or not you can follow the first phase of the Sirt diet will depend on just how thin you already are. While a person who is overweight or well within a healthy weight can practice the first phase, nobody who is clinically underweight should. You can know whether or not you are underweighting by calculating your Body Mass Index, or BMI. You can find many BMI calculators online, and if yours is at nineteen points or below, you should avoid the first phase. It is always a good idea to ask your doctor both if it is safe for you to lose weight, and if the Sirt diet is safe for your individual condition.

While the Sirt diet may generally be safe, for people with certain illnesses, it may not be the case.

While it is understandable to desire to be even more thin, even if you already are thin, pushing yourself past the point of being underweight is incredibly unhealthy, both physically and mentally. This fits into the category of disordered eating and can cause you a lot of harm.

Some of the side effects of pushing your body to extreme weight loss include bone loss and osteoporosis, lowered immune system, fertility problems, and an increased risk of disease. If you want to benefit from the health of the Sirt diet and are underweight, instead consume, however many calories, your doctor recommends, along with plenty of Sirtfoods. This will ensure you maintain a healthy weight while also receiving the benefits that sirtuins have to offer.

If you are thin, but still at a BMI of twenty to twenty-five, then you should be safe beginning the Sirt diet, unless otherwise instructed by your doctor.

Can You Eat Meat and Dairy On The Sirtfood Diet?

In many recipes, we choose to use Sirtfood sources of protein, such as soy, walnuts, and buckwheat. However, this does not mean that you aren't allowed to enjoy meat on the Sirt diet. Sure, it's easy to enjoy a vegan or vegetarian Sirt diet, but if you love your sources of meat, then you don't have to give them up. Protein is an essential aspect of the Sirt diet to preserve muscle tone, and whether you consume only plant-based proteins or a mixture of plant and animal-based proteins is completely up to you. And, just as you can enjoy meat, you can also enjoy moderate consumption of dairy.

Some meats can actually help you better utilize the Sirtfoods you eat. This is because the amino acid leucine can enhance the effect of Sirtfoods. You can find this amino acid in chicken, beef, pork, fish, eggs, dairy, and tofu.

Can I Drink Red Wine during Phase One?

As your calories will be so limited during the first phase, it is not recommended to drink alcohol during this phase. However, you can enjoy it in moderation during phase two and the maintenance phase.

SIRTFOOD FOR BUILDING

MUSCLE

Sirtuins are a group of proteins with different effects. Sirt-1 is the protein responsible for causing the body to burn fat rather than muscle for energy, which is obviously a miracle for weight loss. Another useful aspect of Sirt-1 is its ability to improve skeletal muscle.

Skeletal muscle is all the muscles you voluntarily control, such as the muscles in your limbs, back, shoulders, and so on. There are two other types, cardiac muscle is what the heart is formed of, whilst smooth muscle is your involuntary muscles – which includes muscles around your blood vessels, face, and various parts of organs and other tissues.

Skeletal muscle is separated into two different groups, the blandly named type-1, and type-2. Type 1 muscle is effective at continued, sustained activity whereas type-2 muscle is effective at short, intense periods of activity. So, for example, you would predominantly use type-1 muscles for jogging, but type-2 muscles for sprinting.

Sirt-1 protects the type-1 muscles, but not the type-2 muscle, which is still broken down for energy. Therefore, holistic muscle mass drops when fasting, even though type-1 skeletal muscle mass increases.

Sirt-1 also influences how the muscles actually work. Sirt-1 is produced by the muscle cells, but the ability to produce Sirt-1 decreases as the muscle ages. As a result, muscle is harder to build as you age and doesn't grow as fast in response to exercise. A lack of sirt-1 also causes the muscles to become tired quicker and gradually decline over time.

When you start to consider these effects of Sirt-1, you can start to form a picture of why fasting helps keep the body supple. Fasting releases Sirt-1, which in turn helps skeletal muscle grow and stay in good shape. Sirt-1 is also released by consuming sirtuin activators, giving the Sirtfood diet its muscle retaining power.

Who Should Try the Sirtfood Diet?

The Sirtfood diet is suitable for individuals who:

- Are overweight or obese
- Want to maintain his/her weight
- Needs to have a "detox" and flush away the toxins from the body
- Have failed to lose weight using different diet techniques
- Want not only to lose weight but also build muscle
- Want a healthier lifestyle and to achieve optimal health

Health Risks for Overweight and Obesity

Type 2 Diabetes - This disease occurs when the blood sugar level becomes higher than normal. According to studies, about 80% of individuals afflicted with Type 2 diabetes are overweight. What makes diabetes a killer disease is that it is a major cause of stroke, heart disease, kidney diseases, amputation, and even blindness.

Sleep Apnea - This is when an individual pauses in breathing while sleeping. Being overweight or obese is a risk factor. Why?

This is because of the fats stored in the neck area making the air pathway smaller. Besides, the fat could also cause inflammation.

Sleep apnea should not be taken lightly because it can also result in heart failure.

High Blood Pressure - Also known as hypertension, this condition refers to a state when your systolic blood pressure (usually above 140) is consistently higher than your diastolic blood pressure (usually about 90). How does being overweight make you a high risk for hypertension? Generally, a larger body size will increase your blood pressure so that your heart will have to work harder to produce the necessary supply of blood to all cells. Also, your excess body fats can damage your kidneys (your kidney helps your body regulate blood pressure). High blood pressure can result in kidney failure, heart diseases, and stroke.

Fatty Liver Disease - This is when there is a build-up of fat around the liver which can cause damage.

Reproductive issues - Menstrual issues and ultimately infertility are some of the issues experienced by overweight women.

Cancer - If you are obese or overweight, then the risk of acquiring cancer of the breast, gallbladder, colon, and endometrial increases.

These are only some of the diseases associated with being overweight. Not to mention the social, emotional, and psychological impact of the extra weight.

It stresses the importance of finding the right "strategy" to lose those excess pounds. And we have the perfect solution –the Sirtfood diet.

Are You Familiar with These Scenarios?

You know that you have overindulged during the holidays, but as you weigh yourself, you literally would want to shave all the extra pounds because you did not expect to have gained that much weight!

There is an upcoming wedding event, and you need to lose those extra pounds to fit into your gown/suit. There is no way that you are going to lose that much weight in 2 months!

You know that you are overweight and just plain unhealthy. You have already tried many diets but to no avail. Either you feel that those diets are too restrictive, there is an adverse health effect, and the diet is too expensive to maintain. Speaking of maintenance, you are having a hard time keeping off the little weight that you have managed to lose!

You are getting older and you start to notice that aside from having a hard time dealing with hangovers and late-night parties, losing and maintaining weight is not that easy as it used to be. You are not a big fan of eliminating numerous food groups and doing rigorous exercise.

You have probably heard these scenarios too many times before and you have probably experienced one or two, or you are in one of these scenarios right now. Being overweight or obese is actually one of the most common health problems around the world. According to the World Health Organization (WHO), being overweight is when your BMI is equal to or greater than 25 while being obese is when your BMI is equal to or greater than 30.

In the 2014 data from WHO, worldwide obesity has more than doubled since 1980, and more than 1.9 billion adults are overweight; and it would safe to conclude that after two years that that number has already increased significantly.

Health experts agree that this is a very alarming rate, but the good news is, obesity or having excess weight is preventable and reversible.

As you will notice, most of these scenarios are focused on aesthetics—looking good and feeling more confident about your body, but what I would like to stress is the ill-effects of every extra bulge or pound that we carry. The possible health illnesses associated with being overweight are the primary reason why you need to try the revolutionary SirtFood diet.

BENEFITS OF SIRTFOOD DIET

Fight Fat

The problem with most diets is that once you stop eating them, you will return to your unhealthy eating habits and regain the weight that you are losing. This has happened to many people after stopping their diet.

The real challenge is maintaining your weight if you are satisfied with your weight loss so far.

The Sirtfood diet is also known to control appetite and I don't mean the mind control that fasting encourages. The increase in leptin satisfies us as it reduces our hunger. Makes sense right? Leptin is important as it is the hormone responsible for regulating appetite. This should keep you from asking for more food, but in the case of obesity, leptin may not do its job properly. Due to the hypothalamus, the brain does not feel that the body is well nourished and constantly wants more food, as the brain somehow believes that the body is undernourished. This condition is called leptin resistance.

Build Muscle Mass

When people say they want to lose weight, they are definitely referring to fat loss and not muscle. Fat is lighter than muscle, but we all want to have an optimal BMI, right? There is a myth that a certain amount of protein is needed to maintain muscle mass. Well, that's not entirely true. In the case of fasting, growth hormone reaches incredibly high levels after 72 hours of pure fasting, so you can maintain and even increase your muscle mass due to calorie deprivation. Obviously, it's not healthy to be on a very long fasting

period, but what if you find the right ingredients to eat and have the same benefits?

Obviously, when you are on a high carbohydrate diet you are not building muscle. you are actually accumulating fat. However, the Sirtfood diet is notrich in carbohydrates. It is rich in sirtuins, a very healthy type of protein. The founders of this diet claim that you will lose seven pounds in seven days.

However, food must create the right environment to build or maintain muscle mass, and this is what this diet does. Besides, muscles are important for your mobility and prevent the development of chronic diseases such as osteoporosis or diabetes. Believe it or not, muscles can even have a psychological advantage, as they are known to fight depression. Yes, you willdefinitely feel great about yourself when you look sporty.

SIRT1 is able to maintain muscle mass even when fasting and can even increase your muscle mass. Muscles are made up of various cells, including the satellite cell, which is activated when the muscle is damaged or stressed.

If you do some weight training, basically putting pressure on the muscle, your muscles will grow because of the satellite cell. However, the satellite cell can only be activated by SIRT1. Otherwise, your muscles won't grow, develop, or regenerate properly.

To better comprehend the significance of sirtuins, particularly SIRT1, have in mind that without them your muscles are prone to inflammation and fatigue.

In fact, muscles age without sirtuin activity. Therefore, for muscles to function properly, they really need SIRT1. Muscles do not improve over time, like wine. Keep in mind that the effects of muscle aging can begin at age 25. By the time you reach 40, you have already lost 10 percent of your muscle mass and by the time you are 70, you have already lost 40 percent of your muscle mass. However, this can be prevented and reversed through the activity of sirtuin. Therefore, they can easily be considered as regulators of muscle growth and prevention.

Fight Diseases

The modern-day eating habits and lifestyle encourages the accumulation of fats and toxins (fat tissue protects the toxins), as well as the increase of blood sugar and insulin level. This is where the trouble starts, from a simple prediabetes condition to more serious diseases (it can eventually lead to cancer).

However, the antidote to many of these issues lies hidden within ourselves.

As you already know, all bodies possess sirtuin genes, and activating them is crucial to burn fat and to build a stronger and leaner body.

As it turns out, the benefits of sirtuins activity extend way beyond the fatburning process. Whether we like it or not, the lack of sirtuins can be associated with plenty of diseases and medical conditions. Naturally, activating sirtuins will have the opposite effect. For example, sirtuins can improve your heart health by protecting the muscle cells in your heart and improving the function of the heart muscle. But that's not all. Sirtuins can play a major role in improving the function of your arteries, controlling cholesterol levels, and preventing atherosclerosis.

By now, you are familiar with the effects of fasting and an LCHF diet on the insulin level, and you are probably wondering what sirtuins can do in this case. If you are suffering from diabetes, then you should know that activating sirtuins will make insulin work more effectively to do its job properly (which is regulating the blood sugar level). SIRT1 works perfectly with metformin (one of the most powerful antidiabetic drugs).

As it turns out, pharmaceutical companies are adding sirtuin activators to metformin treatments. These studies were conducted on animals, and the results were simply amazing. It was noticed that an 83 percent reduction of the metformin dose is required to achieve the same effects.

Other diets or programs are bragging about their effects on neurodegenerative diseases, like Alzheimer's disease. Well, let's think about what sirtuins do!

They send a message to the brain, helping it make the right decisions when it comes to appetite suppression. This involves enhancing the communication signals in the brain, improving cognitive function, and lowering brain inflammation. Sirtuin activation stops the tau protein aggregation and amyloid B production, some of the most damaging things in the brains of Alzheimer's patients.

The benefits of sirtuins expand to bones as well, as they encourage the production of osteoblast cells (the ones responsible for strengthening your bones) and increase their survival. In other words, sirtuin activation is very important for overall bone health.

Now, we all know that the food we eat today can even lead to cancer, as we are literally eating small portions of poison. Diets are claiming that they represent the cure for cancer in an incipient form, but at the moment, we can't say this about Sirtfoods, as there are still plenty of studies to be done on this topic. However, it is fair to say that people who eat mostly Sirtfoods have the lowest cancer rates.

Losing weight is simply not enough nowadays, as the diet you have to follow needs to have plenty of health benefits as well; otherwise, you can't stick to it in the long run. Therefore, you need to see the bigger picture and not focus on losing a lot of pounds in a very short amount of time. The less processed food you eat, the more chances you will have to experience the health benefits from your meal plan, so you don't have to see a doctor very often.

Natural ingredients have a lot of vitamins and minerals. They have a very high nutritional value. Coincidence or not, sirtuins can mostly be found in such ingredients (essentially fruits and veggies). Therefore, you will need to unleash these benefits on your body by consuming these amazing ingredients daily.

Anti-Aging Effect

Anti-aging is somehow linked to autophagy, which is an intracellular process of repairing or replacing damaged cell parts. This is rejuvenation at an intracellular level. However, a part of this response is the lysosomal degradation pathway autophagy. Now you are probably wondering what sirtuins have to do with all of these. Well, SIRT1 can activate AMPK (and the other way around), so it can be considered one of the triggers of autophagy. But I'm going to spare you all the chemical details that you can't remember. What you need to know is that autophagy rejuvenates the cell, and this process can happen in all the cells of your body. Starting from the ones of your internal organs to the ones of your skin.

There are a few ways to induce autophagy, and it obviously has a very positive effect on your health and overall lifespan. Just think of the cell as a car and autophagy is the skilled mechanic capable of fixing or replacing any broken parts in it. Obviously, the cell will have a longer life, and this extrapolates to your overall life. If your cells are functioning properly, like a Swiss mechanical clock, then you can expect increased longevity. You can't reverse aging, as there is no such cure for it, and autophagy is not "the fountain of youth." However, this process can significantly slow down aging and its effect. And the best part is that it can be activated by sirtuins, especially SIRT1.

So far, people were not aware of too many ways to trigger autophagy. Some of them were doing it the hard way through intermittent fasting. Others were trying to induce it through an LCHF diet, like the keto diet. Well, now there is an extra way to activate it, and that is through the Sirtfood diet.

Here is a list of other benefits of the Sirtfood Diet:

- Promotes fat loss, not muscle loss
- You will not regain weight after the end of the diet

- You will look better; you will feel better, and you will have more energy
- You will avoid fasting and feeling hungry
- You will not have to undergo exhausting physical exercises

This diet promotes a longer, healthier life and keeps diseases away.

The benefits of the Sirtfood Diet are many, besides obviously that of slimming. Activators of sirtuins would lead to noticeable muscle building, decreased appetite, and improved memory. Also, the Sirtfood Diet normalizes the level of sugar in the blood and can cleanse the cells from the accumulation of harmful free radicals.

MAIN DISHES

Green Beans With Crispy Chickpeas

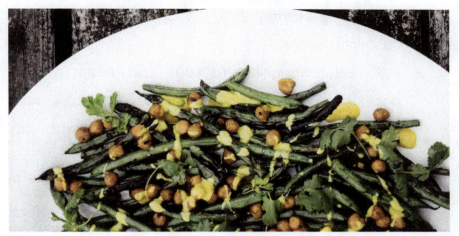

Preparation Time: **30 minutes**

Cooking Time: **10 minutes**

Servings: **4**

Ingredients:

- 1 can chickpeas, rinsed
- 1 tsp. whole coriander
- 1 lb. green beans, trimmed
- 2 tbsp. olive oil, divided
- Kosher salt and freshly ground black pepper
- 1 tsp. cumin seeds
- Grilled lemons, for serving

Directions
1. Heat grill to medium. Gather chickpeas, coriander, cumin, and 1 tbsp. oil in a medium cast-iron skillet.
2. Put skillet on grill and cook chickpeas, mixing occasionally, until golden brown and coriander begins to pop, 5 to 6 minutes. Season with salt and pepper.
3. Transfer to a bowl.
4. Add green beans and remaining tbsp. olive oil to the skillet.
5. Add salt and pepper.
6. Cook, turning once, until charred and barely tender, 3 to 4 minutes. Toss green beans with chickpea mixture and serve with grilled lemons alongside.

Nutrition Facts: **Calories: 460 Fat: 15g Carbs: 57g Protein: 16g**

Sloppy Joe Scramble Stuffed Spuds

Preparation Time: **25 minutes**

Cooking Time: **50 minutes**

Servings: **6 potato halves**

Ingredients:
- 1 tbsp. high heat neutral-flavored oil
- 1 pound extra-firm tofu, drained, pressed, and crumbled
- ¼ tsp fine sea salt
- ¼ tsp ground black pepper
- ¾ cup onion, finely chopped
- ¼ cup bell pepper (any color), finely chopped
- 3 cloves garlic, finely chopped
- 1 tbsp. ground cumin
- 2 tsp chili powder, or to taste
- 1 can (15 oz.) tomato sauce
- 2 tbsp. organic ketchup
- 1 tbsp. tamari
- 1 tbsp. Worcestershire sauce
- 1 tbsp. yellow mustard
- 1 4-inch dill pickle, minced
- ¾ cup water
- 3 baked potatoes, cooled
- 1 tbsp. olive oil

Directions:
1. Heat 1 tbsp. of oil in a large skillet over medium-high heat.
2. If the skillet is not well-seasoned, add the remaining tbsp. of oil. Add the tofu, salt, and pepper. Cook for 8 to 10 minutes, occasionally stirring until the tofu is firm and golden.
3. Stir in the onion, bell pepper, garlic, cumin, and chili powder.
4. Reduce the heat to medium and cook for 3 minutes, occasionally stirring, until fragrant.
5. Add the tomato sauce, ketchup, tamari, Worcestershire sauce, mustard, and dill pickle.
6. Bring to a boil, and then reduce the heat to simmer. Swish the water in the tomato sauce can to clean the sides.
7. Simmer for 30 minutes, occasionally stirring, adding the water from the tomato sauce can.
8. As needed for the desired consistency.
9. Preheat the oven to broil.
10. Cut the baked potatoes in half lengthwise.
11. Scoop the insides from the potatoes, leaving about 1 inch of the skin intact.

12. Brush both the insides and the outsides of the potato skins with the olive oil and place them on a baking sheet. Broil for 3 to 4 minutes until lightly browned.
13. Remove from the oven and divide the filling evenly in the potatoes, using about ¼ cup in each.

Nutrition Facts: Calories: 306 Fat: 21g Carbohydrate: 6g Protein: 23g

Baked Salmon Salad With Creamy Mint Dressing

Preparation Time: **20 minutes**

Cooking Time: **25 minutes**

Servings: **1**

Ingredients:

- 1 salmon fillet
- 1 cup mixed salad leaves
- 1 cup lettuce leaves
- Two radishes, thinly sliced
- ½ cucumber, sliced
- 2 spring onions, trimmed and chopped
- ½ oz. parsley, roughly sliced
- For the dressing:
- 1 tsp low-carb mayonnaise
- 1 tbsp. natural yogurt
- 1 tbsp. rice vinegar
- 2 stalks mint, finely chopped

Directions:

1. Put the salmon fillet onto a baking tray and bake for 16--18 minutes until cooked in a bowl, blend together the mayonnaise, yogurt, rice vinegar, mint leaves and salt and set aside 5 minutes to the flavors to mix well.

2. Arrange the salad leaves and lettuce onto a serving plate and top with all the radishes, cucumber, lettuce, celery, spring onions and parsley.
3. Drizzle the dressing.

Nutrition Facts: Calories: 433 Fat: 9g Carbohydrate: 32g Protein: 18g

Fragrant Asian Hot Pot

Preparation Time: **15 minutes**

Cooking Time: **25 minutes**

Servings: **2**

Ingredients:
- 1 tsp tomato purée
- 1 star anise, crushed
- ½ oz. parsley, finely chopped
- ½ oz. coriander, finely chopped
- Juice of 1/2 lime
- 2 cups chicken stock
- ½ carrot, cut into matchsticks
- ½ cup cauliflower cut into small florets
- 2oz beansprouts
- 4oz raw tiger prawns
- 2oz rice noodles, cooked as per packet directions
- 2oz cooked water chestnuts, drained
- 20g sushi ginger, sliced
- 1 tbsp. high miso paste

Directions:
1. Set the tomato purée, star anise, parsley stalks, coriander stalks, lime juice and chicken stock in a large pan and bring to a simmer for about 10 minutes.

2. Add the beansprouts, cauliflower, carrot, prawns, tofu, noodles and water chestnuts and simmer gently until the prawns are cooked.
3. Remove from the heat and stir at the skillet along with miso paste. Serve sprinkled with the parsley and coriander leaves.

Nutrition Facts: Calories: 397 Fat: 15g Carbohydrate: 33g Protein: 19g

Tofu Scramble With Mushrooms

Preparation Time: **15 minutes**

Cooking Time: **10 minutes**

Servings: **2**

Ingredients:

- 3 tbsp. olive oil
- ½ yellow onion, diced
- 3 cloves garlic, finely chopped
- 1 tsp. soy sauce
- 12oz firm tofu, cubed
- ½ red bell pepper, diced
- ¾ cup mushrooms, cut
- 3 green onions, diced
- 2 tomatoes, cleaved
- ½ tsp. ground ginger
- ½ tsp. bean stew powder
- ¼ tsp. cayenne pepper
- Salt and pepper to taste

Directions:

1. Gently sauté onion and garlic in the olive oil for 3 to 5 minutes, until they are soft.
2. Add the remaining ingredients, except salt and pepper.

3. Sautee for another 6 to 8 minutes, until veggies are done and tofu absorbed the liquid.
4. Add salt and pepper, to taste.

Nutrition Facts: Calories: 330 Fat: 9g Carbohydrate: 36g Protein: 18g

Prawn Arrabbiata

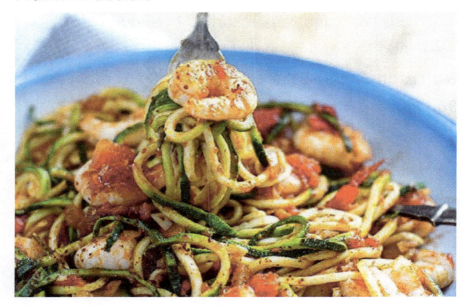

Preparation Time: **40 minutes**

Cooking Time: **60 minutes**

Servings: **1**

Ingredients:

- 5oz raw prawns
- 2oz Buckwheat pasta
- 1 tbsp. extra virgin olive oil
- ½ Red onion, finely chopped
- 1 Garlic clove, finely chopped
- 1oz Celery, thinly sliced
- 1 Bird's eye chili, thinly sliced
- 1 tsp Dried mixed herbs
- 1 tsp extra virgin olive oil

- 2 tbsp. White wine
- ½ tin chopped tomatoes
- 1 tbsp. Chopped parsley

Directions:

1. Fry the garlic, onion, celery and herbs in oil over low heat for 1-2 minutes.
2. Raise the heat to medium, add the wine and cook until it has evaporated Add the tomatoes and let the sauce cook for 20-30 minutes, until it is reduced and has a rich texture.
3. While the sauce is cooking, bring a little water to a boil and cook the pasta as indicated on the package.
4. When cooked, drain and set aside.
5. Place the shrimp in the sauce and cook for another 3-4 minutes, until they are opaque and pink, then add the parsley and cooked pasta to the sauce, mix and serve.

Nutrition Facts: Calories: 335 Fat: 12g Carbohydrate: 38g Protein: 19g

Turmeric Baked Salmon

Preparation Time: **15 minutes**

Cooking Time: **30 minutes**

Servings: **1**

Ingredients:

- 6 oz. Salmon fillet, skinned
- 1 tsp. extra virgin olive oil
- 1 tsp. Ground turmeric
- ¼ lemon, juiced

For the sauce:

- 1 tsp. extra virgin olive oil
- 1 oz. Red onion, finely chopped
- 1 oz. Tinned green peas
- 1 Garlic clove, finely chopped
- 1-inch fresh ginger, finely chopped
- 1 Bird's eye chili, thinly sliced
- 4 oz. Celery cut into small cubes
- 1 tsp Mild curry powder
- 1 Tomato, chopped
- ½ cup vegetable stock
- 1 tbsp. parsley, chopped

Directions:

1. Heat the oven to 400 ° F. Begin to cook the sauce. Heat a skillet over medium heat, then add

the olive oil, garlic, onion, ginger, chilli and celery.
2. Stir lightly for 2-3 minutes until soft but not colored, then add the curry powder and cook for another minute.
3. Add the tomato, peas and broth and cook for 10/15 minutes depending on how thick you like the sauce.
4. Meanwhile, combine the turmeric, oil and lemon juice and rub the salmon.
5. Place on a baking sheet and bake for 10 minutes in the oven. Serve the salmon with the celery sauce.

Nutrition Facts: Calories: 360 Fat: 8g Carbs: 10g Protein: 40g

Baked Potatoes With Spicy Chickpea Stew

Preparation Time: **10 minutes**

Cooking Time: **60 minutes**

Servings: **4**

Ingredients:

- 4 baking potatoes, pricked around
- 2 tbsp. olive oil
- 2 red onions, finely chopped
- 4 tsp. garlic, crushed or grated
- 1-inch ginger, grated
- 1/2 tsp chili flakes
- 2 tbsp. cumin seeds
- 2 tbsp. turmeric
- Splash of water
- 2 tins chopped tomatoes
- 2 tbsp. cocoa powder, unsweetened
- 2 tins chickpeas – do not drain
- 2 yellow peppers, chopped
- 2 tbsp.

Directions:

1. Preheat the oven to 400F; and start preparing all the ingredients. When the oven is ready, place the potatoes in the oven and cook for 50min-1 hour until ready.

2. While the potatoes are cooking, place the olive oil and sliced red onion in a large, wide saucepan and cook lightly, covering, for 5 minutes until the onions are tender but not golden. Remove the lid and add the ginger, garlic, cumin and cook for another minute over very low heat.
3. Then add the turmeric and some water and cook for a few more minutes until it becomes thicker and the consistency is ok.
4. Then add the tomatoes, cocoa powder, peppers, chickpeas with their water and salt.
5. Bring to a boil and then cook over very low heat for 45-50 minutes until thick.
6. Finally incorporate the 2 tbsp. parsley, pepper and salt if you wish, and also serve the stew with potatoes.

Nutrition Facts: Calories: 520 Fat: 8g Carbohydrate: 91g Protein: 32g

Kale And Red Onion Dhal With Buckwheat

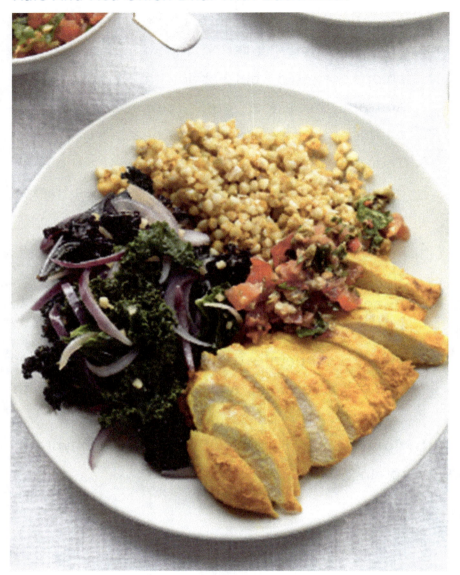

Preparation Time: **5 minutes**

Cooking Time: **35 minutes**

Servings: **4**

Ingredients:
- 1 tbsp. olive oil
- 1 small red onion, sliced
- 3 garlic cloves, crushed or grated
- 2-inch ginger, grated
- 1 bird's eye chili deseeded, chopped
- 2 tsp. turmeric
- 2 tsp. garam masala
- 6oz snow peas
- 2 cups coconut milk, unsweetened
- 1 cup water
- 1 cup carrot, thinly sliced
- 6oz buckwheat

Directions:
1. Put the olive oil in a large, deep pan and then add the chopped onion.
2. Cook over low heat, with the lid on for 5 minutes, until softened.
3. Add the ginger, garlic and chilli and cook 1 minute.
4. Add the turmeric and garam masala along with a drop of water and cook for 1 minute.

5. Add the snow peas, coconut milk, and 1 cup of water. Mix everything together and cook for 20 minutes on low heat with the lid on.
6. Stir occasionally and add a little more water if the dhal starts to stick.
7. After 20 minutes add the carrot, mix well and cook for another 5 minutes.
8. While the dhal is cooking, steam the buckwheat in boiling salted water for 15 minutes, drain and serve with the dhal.

Nutrition Facts: Calories: 340 Fat: 4g Carbohydrate: 30g Protein: 4g

Kale, Edamame And Tofu Curry

Preparation Time: **30 minutes**

Cooking Time: **45 minutes**

Servings: **4**

Ingredients:
- 1 tbsp. oil
- 1 big onion, chopped
- 4 cloves garlic, peeled and grated
- 1 3-inch fresh ginger, peeled and grated
- 1 red chili, deseeded and thinly sliced
- 1/2 tsp. ground turmeric
- 1/4 tsp. cayenne pepper
- 1 tsp. paprika
- 1/2 tsp. ground cumin
- 1 tsp. salt
- 8 oz. dried red lentils
- 2 oz. soya edamame beans
- 8 oz. firm tofu, cubed
- 2 tomatoes, roughly chopped
- Juice of 1 lime
- ½ cup parsley, stalks removed

Directions:
1. Put the oil in a pan over medium heat. When the oil is hot, add the onion and cook for 5 minutes.

2. Add the ginger, garlic and chilli and cook for another 2 minutes.
3. Add the turmeric, cayenne pepper, paprika, cumin and salt.
4. Mix and add the red lentils, edamame soy beans and tomatoes.
5. Pour in 4 cups of boiling water and then bring to a boil for about 10 minutes, then lower the heat and cook for another 40 minutes until the curry thickens and all the flavors have blended.
6. Add the lime juice and parsley, mix and serve.

Nutrition Facts: Calories: 325 Fat: 6g Carbs: 77g Protein: 28g

Lemon Chicken With Spinach, Red Onion, And Salsa

Preparation Time: **30 minutes**

Cooking Time: **35 minutes**

Servings: **1**

Ingredients:

- 4oz chicken breast, skinless, boneless
- 1 large tomato
- 1 chili, finely chopped
- 1oz capers
- Juice of 1/2 lemon
- 2 tbsp. extra-virgin olive oil
- 2 cups spinach
- 20g red onion, chopped
- 2 tsp chopped garlic
- 3oz buckwheat

Directions:

1. Heat the oven to 400 ° F.
2. To make the sauce, chop the tomato very finely and place it with its liquid in a bowl.
3. The liquid is very important because it is very tasty.
4. Mix with chilli, capers, onion, 1 tablespoon of oil and a few drops of lemon juice.

5. Marinate the chicken breast with garlic, lemon juice and ½ tablespoon of oil for 10 minutes.
6. Heat an ovenproof skillet until hot, add the chicken and cook for one minute on each side, until golden brown, then bake (put on a baking sheet if the pan is not ovenproof) for 5 minutes until cooked. Remove from the oven and cover with aluminum foil.
7. Leave to rest for 5 minutes before serving.
8. Meanwhile, sauté the spinach for 5 minutes with ½ tablespoon of oil and 1 tablespoon of garlic.
9. It goes well with chicken with sauce and spinach.

Nutrition Facts: Calories: 342 Fat: 8g Carbs: 18g Protein: 33g

Smoked Salmon Omelet

Preparation Time: **10 minutes**

Cooking Time: **15 minutes**

Servings: **1**

Ingredients:
- 2 eggs
- 4oz Smoked salmon, chopped
- 1/2 tsp. Capers
- ½ cup Rocket, chopped
- 1 tsp Parsley, chopped
- 1 tsp extra virgin olive oil

Directions:
1. Break the eggs into a bowl and beat well. Add the salmon, capers, rocket and parsley.
2. Heat the olive oil in a pan.
3. Add the egg mixture and, with a spatula, move the mixture around the pan until it is uniform.
4. Lower the heat and let the omelette cook.
5. Turn the spatula around the edges to lift them, add the salmon and rocket and fold the omelette in 2.

Facts: Calories: 303 Fat: 22g Carbohydrate: 12g Protein: 23g

Broccoli And Pasta

Preparation Time: **20 minutes**

Cooking Time: **10 minutes**

Servings: **2**

Ingredients:
- 5 oz. spaghetti
- 5 oz. broccoli
- 1 garlic clove, finely chopped
- 3 tbsp. extra virgin olive oil
- 2 Shallots sliced
- ¼ tsp. crushed chilies
- 12 sage shredded leaves
- Grated parmesan (optional)

Directions:
1. Put the broccoli in boiling water for 5 minutes, then add the spaghetti and cook until the pasta and broccoli are cooked (about 8-10 minutes).
2. Meanwhile, heat the oil in a pan and add the shallot and garlic. Cook for 5 minutes until golden.
3. Mix the chillies and sage in the pan and cook gently for more than 1 minute.
4. Drain pasta and broccoli; mix with the pan-fried shallot mixture, add some Parmesan if desired and serve.

Nutrition Facts: Calories: 350 Fat: 8g Carbs: 38g Protein: 6g

Artichokes and Kale with Walnuts

Preparation Time: **10 minutes**

Cooking Time: **30 minutes**

Servings: **2**

Ingredients:

- 1 cup of artichoke hearts
- 1 tbsp. parsley, chopped
- ½ cup of walnuts
- 1 cup of kale, torn
- 1 cup of Cheddar cheese, crumbled
- ½ tbsp. balsamic vinegar
- 1 tbsp. olive oil
- Salt and black pepper, to taste

Directions:

1. Preheat the oven to 250°-270° Fahrenheit and roast the nuts in the oven for 10 minutes until lightly browned and crisp, then set aside.
2. Add the artichoke hearts, kale, oil, salt and pepper to a saucepan and cook for 20-25 minutes until done.
3. Add the cheese and balsamic vinegar and mix well.
4. Divide the vegetables into two plates and garnish with toasted nuts and parsley.

Nutrition Facts: Calories: 152 kcal; Fat: 32g; Carbohydrates: 59g; Protein: 23g

Pecan Crusted Chicken Breast

Preparation Time: **20 minutes**

Cooking Time: **35 minutes**

Servings: **4**

Ingredients:
- ½ cup whole wheat bread, dried
- 1/3 cup pecans
- 2 tbsp. Parmesan
- Salt and ground pepper
- 1 egg white
- 4 chicken breasts slices, boneless and skinless (6 to 8 oz. each)
- 1 tbsp. grapeseed oil
- Lemon cuts, for serving
- 1 cup mixed greens
- 1tbsp olive oil

Directions:
1. Preheat the oven to 425 ° F. In a food processor, blitz bread, pecans and parmesan; season with salt and pepper until you get a thin breadcrumbs.
2. Move to a bowl. In another bowl, beat the egg white until fluffy. Season the chicken with salt and pepper.

3. Sprinkle each slice of chicken breast with egg white first, then place it in the bowl of breadcrumbs and mix until completely covered. In a large non-stick pan, heat the grapeseed oil over medium heat.
4. When hot, place the chicken breasts to cook until lightly seared, 1 to 3 minutes.
5. Flip the chicken over and place the pan in the oven.
6. Cook until the chicken is cooked through (about 8-12 minutes). Serve the chicken with lemon slices and a plate of mixed vegetables with olive oil, lemon and salt.

Nutrition Facts: Calories: 250 Fat: 8g Carbohydrates: 27g Protein: 17g

Tuna And Tomatoes

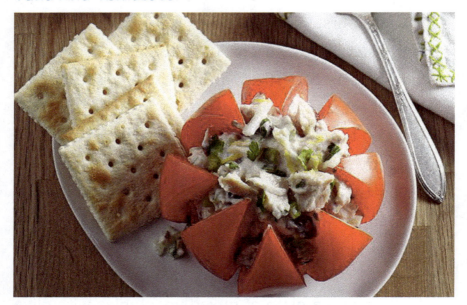

Preparation Time: **5 minutes**

Cooking Time: **20 minutes**

Servings: **4**

Ingredients:

- 1 yellow onion, chopped
- 1 tbsp. olive oil
- 1 lb. tuna fillets, skinless and cubed
- 1 cup tomatoes, chopped
- 1 red pepper, chopped
- 1 tsp sweet paprika
- 1 tbsp. coriander, chopped

Directions:

1. Heat a pan with oil over medium heat, add the onions and pepper and cook for 5 minutes, they must be crunchy and crunchy: do not overcook.
2. Add the tuna, tomato and paprika and cook quickly 1 minute over high heat.
3. Add the coriander and serve immediately.

Nutrition Facts: Calories 215 kcal, Fat 4g, Carbs 14g, Protein 7g

Tuna And Kale

Preparation Time: **5 minutes**

Cooking Time: **20 minutes**

Servings: **4**

Ingredients:

- 1lb tuna fillets, skinless and cubed
- A pinch of salt and black pepper
- 2 tbsp. olive oil
- 1 cup kale
- ½ cup cherry tomatoes, cubed
- 1 yellow onion, chopped

Directions:

1. Steam the black cabbage for 6 minutes, season 1 tablespoon of olive and a pinch of salt and mix well.
2. Heat a skillet with the remaining oil over medium heat; add the onion and brown for 5 minutes.
3. Add the tuna and cherry tomatoes and cook for 5 minutes.
4. Serve the tuna with the black cabbage on the side.

Nutrition Facts: Calories 251 kcal, Fat 4g, Carbohydrate 14g, Protein 7g

Salmon & Kale Omelet

Preparation Time: **10 minutes**

Cooking Time: **7 minutes**

Servings: **4**

Ingredients:
- 6 eggs
- 2 tbsp. almond milk, unsweetened
- Salt and ground black pepper, to taste
- 2 tbsp. olive oil
- 4 oz. smoked salmon, cut into bite-sized chunks
- 2 cup fresh kale, tough ribs removed and chopped finely
- 4 scallions, chopped finely

Directions:
1. In a bowl, put the eggs, almond milk, salt and black pepper and mix well. To put aside.
2. In a nonstick skillet, heat the oil over medium heat.
3. Put a tablespoon of egg mixture, distribute it evenly by turning the pan and cook for about 1 minute.
4. Spread the salmon cabbage and shallot evenly over the egg mixture. Reduce the heat to low and

cook for about 4-5 minutes, or until the omelette is completely cooked.
5. Carefully, transfer the omelette to a serving dish and serve.

Nutrition Facts: Calories 210 kcal Fat 14.9 g Carbohydrates 5.2 g Protein 14.8 g

Moroccan Spiced Eggs

Preparation Time: **1 hour**

Cooking Time: **50 minutes**

Servings: **2**

Ingredients:
- 1 tsp. olive oil
- 1 shallot, finely chopped
- 1 red bell pepper, finely chopped
- 1 garlic clove, finely chopped
- 1 zucchini, finely chopped
- 1 tbsp. tomato paste
- ½ tsp. mild curry
- ¼ tsp. ground cinnamon
- ¼ tsp. ground cumin
- ½ tsp. salt
- 1 can tomatoes
- 1 can chickpeas, drained
- 1/3oz parsley
- 4 medium eggs at room temperature

Directions:
1. Heat the oil in a pan; Include the shallot and red pepper and sauté over low heat for 5 minutes.
2. Add the garlic and zucchini and cook for 2 minutes.

3. Add the tomato paste, spices and salt and mix well.
4. Add the tomatoes and chickpeas and bring to medium heat.
5. Cover and simmer for 30 minutes until it becomes thicker. R
6. emove from the heat and add the chopped parsley.
7. Preheat the grill to 350F. Put the tomato sauce in a pan and break the eggs in the center.
8. Place the pan under the grill for 10 minutes and serve.

Nutrition Facts: Calories: 316 kcal Fat: 5.22 g Carbohydrates: 13.14 g, Protein: 6.97 g

Chickpea, Quinoa And Turmeric Curry Recipe

Preparation Time: **10 minutes**

Cooking Time: **1 hour**

Servings: **4**

Ingredients:

- 1lb potatoes
- 3 garlic cloves, squashed
- 3 tsp ground turmeric
- 1 tsp ground coriander
- 1 tsp mild curry
- 1 tsp ground ginger
- 2 cups coconut milk, unsweetened
- 1 tbsp. tomato purée
- 1 can of tomatoes
- 6oz quinoa
- 1 can chickpeas, drained
- 2 cups spinach

Directions:

1. Put the potatoes in a pan, covered with cold water and bring to a boil, then cook for 25 minutes are soft (always check with a stick). Drain them well, remove the skin and set aside.

2. Put the garlic, turmeric, coriander, bean stew, ginger, coconut milk, tomato puree and tomatoes in a pan.
3. Bring to the boil, season with salt and pepper; then include the quinoa with another glass of water.
4. Put on low heat, put a lid on and let it simmer for 30 minutes, stirring occasionally.
5. Halfway through cooking, add the chickpeas. When there are only 5 minutes left, add the spinach and coarsely chopped potatoes.
6. Divide into 4 portions and serve immediately.

Nutrition Facts: Calories: 609 kcal Fat: 12.15 g Carbohydrates: 85.27, Protein: 23.04 g

Chili Sweetcorn And Wild Garlic Fritters

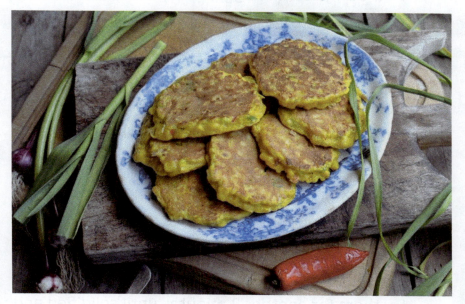

Preparation Time: **5 min**

Cooking Time: **10 min**

Servings: **4**

Ingredients:

- ¾ cup Self-rising flour
- 2 cups Tinned or frozen sweetcorn
- 3 Medium free-range eggs
- 1 Red chili, finely chopped
- Fry-light extra virgin olive oil spray
- ¾ cup Wild garlic leaves and bulbs, finely diced
- 2 cups lettuce, chopped

Direction:

1. In a bowl, mix the eggs, flour, chilli, diced bear's garlic and sweet corn, season with pepper and salt.
2. Spray a large non-stick pan and put it over medium heat.
3. Use a spoon to pour the egg mixture into the pan, batch by batch.
4. The mixture will give you two large pancakes per person or four small pancakes.
5. Fry the pancakes for about four minutes on one side, then turn them gently on the other side and fry them for another 3 minutes until solidified and golden.
6. Serve immediately with salad.

Nutrition Facts: Calories: 198 Fat: 7g Carbohydrates: 30g Protein: 3g

Roast Mackerel And Simple Veggies

Preparation Time: **5 min**

Cooking Time: **25 min**

Servings: **4**

Ingredients:
- 2oz Pitted black olives
- 2 Leeks, chopped
- 7oz Cherry tomatoes
- 2 Sweet potatoes, chopped
- 1tbsp extra virgin olive oil
- 1 Lemon, juiced
- 11oz Mackerel fillets
- ¼ pint Vegetable stock

Directions:
1. Preheat the oven to 375 degrees F.
2. Place the chopped leeks and sweet potatoes in a baking dish.
3. Pour over the vegetable broth and drizzle with extra virgin olive oil. Place the pan in the oven to roast for about 15-20 minutes.
4. Remove from the oven, add the black olives, cherry tomatoes and mackerel fillets, then squeeze the lemon juice all over.
5. Return to the oven to roast another 10 minutes.

6. It is needed immediately.

Nutrition Facts: Calories: 374 Fat: 12g Carbohydrate: 48g Protein: 17g

Baked Root Veg With Chili

Preparation Time: **20 minutes**

Cooking Time: **50 minutes**

Servings: **4**

Ingredients:

- 3 medium Potatoes
- 3 medium Sweet potatoes
- 3 small Yam
- 2 cups Vegetable broth
- 1 can Red kidney beans
- 1 can White kidney beans
- 2 cans Diced tomatoes
- 1 can Black beans
- 1 tbsp. Dried oregano
- 2 tbsp. Paprika
- 1 tsp Cumin
- 2 tsp Chili powder
- 2 stalks Celery
- 2 medium Carrots
- 1 Bell pepper
- 2 Red onions
- 3 tbsp. Olive oil
- ½ oz. Cilantro
- 2 Avocados

- 1 Bay leaf
- 1 can Sweet corn
- 2 Tomatoes
- 2 Limes, juiced
- 1 head Romaine

Directions:

1. Scrub and fork the potatoes and yams.
2. Season them with the oil.
3. Sprinkle with salt and place on a baking sheet for 45 minutes or until you can prick easily with a knife.
4. Heat the oil in a skillet over medium heat and add the diced onion with the chopped pepper, diced carrots and celery along with a quarter teaspoon of salt.
5. Cook until the carrot is tender, then add the paprika, oregano, cumin, and chili powder.
6. Add the tomato, bay leaf and vegetable broth.
7. Rinse the beans and drain them well before adding them to the pot.
8. Mix well and let it simmer for another 30 minutes.

9. After this time, get yourself a potato masher and mash the chilli a few times to crush part of the beans and thicken the mixture.
10. Add the juice of a lime and season with salt and pepper.
11. In a bowl, finely say the avocado and lightly mash it with salt, pepper and the juice of another lime.
12. In another bowl, drain and rinse the corn and season with the cilantro, finely chopped romaine lettuce, a pinch of salt and a spoon. Olive oil.
13. Serve potatoes, chili, avocado and salad so that everyone can assemble their own masterpiece. To enjoy!

Nutrition Facts: Calories: 493kcal; Fat: 14g; Carbohydrates: 96g Protein:14g;

Autumn Stuffed Enchiladas

Preparation Time: **35 minutes**

Cooking Time: **50 minutes**

Servings: **2**

Ingredients:

- 1 Lemon, juiced
- 1 cup raw Cashews
- ½ oz. Cilantro
- 1 oz. Roasted pumpkin seeds
- 12 Corn tortillas
- 2 cups Butternut squash
- 1 cup Salsa
- 1 can Black beans
- 2 tbsp. Olive oil
- ¼ tbsp. Cayenne pepper
- 1 tsp Chili flakes
- 1 tsp Cumin
- 3 cloves Garlic
- 1 Jalapeno
- 1 Red onion
- 1 cup Brussel sprouts

Directions:

1. Soak the cashews in boiling water and set aside.

2. Cut the pumpkin in half and after collecting the seeds;
3. Lightly rub the olive oil. Sprinkle with some salt and pepper before placing on a face-down baking sheet.
4. Cook for about forty-five minutes at 400F until cooked.
5. Heat a spoon. olive oil in a skillet over medium heat and put the chopped onion, stirring until soft.
6. Finely chop the jalapeño and garlic and finely slice the Brussels sprouts.
7. Add these three things to the pan and cook until the Brussels starts to wilt.
8. Strain and rinse the black beans then add them to the pan and mix well. When the squash is cooked and cold enough to handle, scrape the soft insides off the skin and place it in a large bowl along with the Brussels mixture.
9. Mix well again with salt and pepper to taste. Put the tortillas in the oven to soften (don't make them crunchy) Pour the pumpkin mixture into the center of the soft tortillas.

10. Roll them up carefully to make small open wraps, then place them on a baking sheet with the open ends down to prevent them from unrolling.
11. Do this for all twelve tortillas, then pour in the rest of the sauce and distribute it evenly.
12. Change the oven temperature to 350F and bake for 30 minutes. While these cooks put the drained and soaked cashews in a blender with one and a half cups of cold water, lemon juice and a quarter teaspoon of salt.
13. Blend until the mixture is smooth, adding water if it becomes too thick.
14. This is your sour cream. When the enchiladas are ready, let them cool while you chop the cilantro.
15. Then generously pour the sour cream onto the plate and garnish with cilantro and pumpkin seeds.

Nutrition Facts: Calories: 333kcal; Fat: 11g Carbohydrate: 36g; Protein: 14g;

Creamy Vegetable Casserole

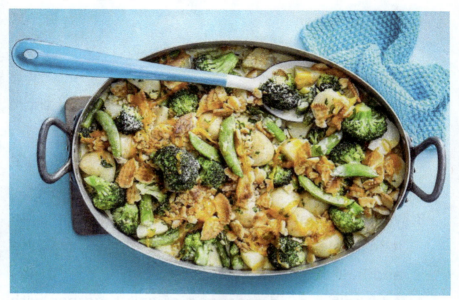

Preparation Time: **30 minutes**

Cooking Time: **60 minutes**

Servings: **2**

Ingredients:
- 2 tbsp. Fresh rosemary
- 1 tsp Dried basil
- 1tsp Dried oregano
- 3 cloves Garlic
- ¼ cup Nutritional yeast
- 2tbsp Olive oil
- 2 tbsp. Apple cider vinegar
- 1 cup raw cashews
- 2 Zucchini

- 1 stalk Broccoli
- 1 Cauliflower
- 10 Russet potatoes

Directions:
1. Pour boiled water over the cashews and let them soak.
2. Cut the cauliflower into small florets and boil it until soft.
3. When the cauliflower is cooked, drain it and put it in a blender along with the drained cashews and half a glass of cold water.
4. Add half a good teaspoon of salt together with the apple cider vinegar and nutritional yeast.
5. Blend until creamy.
6. Wash and grate the courgettes, set them aside.
7. Cut the broccoli into small pieces and set aside.
8. Sprinkle the sides and bottom of a baking sheet with olive oil.
9. Cut the potatoes as thin as possible and spread them out in the pan forming an even layer.
10. Pour in half of the cauliflower sauce to cover and distribute evenly. Add the grated zucchini and spread to cover the sauce.

11. Sprinkle the oregano and basil over the zucchini, then insert the broccoli pieces into the zucchini to keep the surface as even as possible.
12. Drizzle some more cauliflower sauce around the broccoli pieces to fill in the gaps.
13. Make another layer to use the rest of the potatoes, then pour the rest of the remaining cauliflower sauce on top. Spread it out as evenly as possible, right up to the edges to fill in all the spaces around the sides. Sprinkle the top with half a teaspoon of black pepper and a generous pinch or two of salt. Finely chop the fresh rosemary and sprinkle it on top.
14. Bake at 400F for 45 minutes.
15. It will be done when a knife pierces the potatoes without picking them up and the top should be golden brown.
16. Let it cool before serving.

Nutrition Facts: Calories: 389kcal; Fat: 4g; Carbohydrate: 37g; Protein: 26g

Vegan Mac And Cheese

Preparation Time: **25 minutes**

Cooking Time: **30 minutes**

Servings: **2**

Ingredients:

- 1 cup raw Cashews
- ½ tsp Chili flakes
- ½ cup Nutritional yeast
- Salt and pepper to taste
- ½ tsp mustard powder
- ½ tsp Onion powder
- ½ tsp Garlic powder
- 3 cloves Garlic
- 1 Russet potato
- 1 White onion
- 2tbsp Avocado oil
- 1 head Broccoli
- 1 ½ tsp Apple cider vinegar
- 2 cups Macaroni

Directions:

1. Peel and grate the potato.
2. Finely says garlic. Heat a large saucepan and oil over medium heat.

3. Put the onion and some salt into the pot and cook until soft.
4. Add the potato, chili, garlic, mustard, onion, and garlic powders to the pot. Mix well until their flavors release, then add a cup of water and cashews.
5. Continue stirring over a low heat until the potatoes are soft. Pour the entire mixture into a blender along with the apple cider vinegar and nutritional yeast, salt and pepper.
6. The consistency should be that of the cheese sauce which is thick but runny.
7. If it is too thick, add more water, if it needs more salt or garlic powder, red pepper flakes or vinegar, do it now to your taste.
8. Boil the pasta in abundant salted water.
9. In another pot, boil the broccoli in small flowers until tender.
10. When both are ready, transfer everything to a saucepan and cover with the cheese sauce.
11. Combine well, serve and enjoy your meal!

Nutrition Facts: Calories: 263kcal; Fat: 14g; carbohydrates: 36g; Protein: 4g;

Butternut Squash Alfredo

Preparation Time: **15 minutes**

Cooking Time: **25 minutes**

Servings: **4**

Ingredients:

- 9oz Whole grain linguine
- 2 cups Vegetable broth
- 3 cups Butternut Squash, diced
- Salt and pepper to taste
- 1 tsp Paprika
- 2 cloves Garlic
- 1 White onion
- 1 cup Green peas
- 1 Zucchini
- 2tbsp Olive oil
- 2 tbsp. Sage

Directions:

1. Heat the oil in a large skillet over medium heat.
2. As it heats up, make sure the sage leaves are clean and dry, then put them in the oil to fry, moving so as not to burn.
3. Take them out and place them on a paper towel.

4. In the pan, place the peeled and diced pumpkin along with the paprika, diced onion and black pepper.
5. Cook until the onion is soft, then add the broth and season with salt. Bring to a boil before lowering the heat and allowing the pumpkin to cook.
6. In another pot, cook the linguine in water with a little salt. When the squash is tender, put it in a blender along with all the liquid and other ingredients.
7. Blend until creamy and taste to see if you need more salt, pepper, or spices.
8. Return it to the pan to keep it warm over low heat.
9. Using a grater, grate the zucchini lengthwise to obtain long noodles.
10. Make them as long as you can to blend in with the linguine.
11. Add them to the sauce along with the peas and cook in the pumpkin for five minutes.
12. When the pasta is ready, save a cup of liquid before draining it.

13. Add the linguine to the pasta and mix well to coat the linguine.
14. If the sauce is too thick, add a little water to the pasta.
15. Serve the pasta topped with the fried sage leaves and a little black pepper.

Nutrition Facts: Calories: 432; Fat: 14g; Carbohydrate: 36g; Protein: 34g;

Cajun Turkey Rice

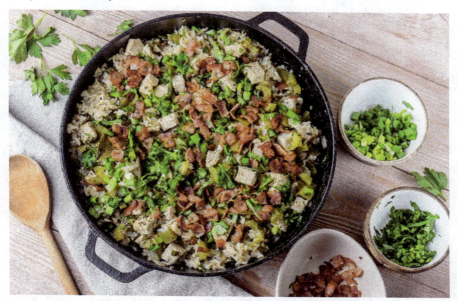

Preparation Time: **10 minutes**

Cooking Time: **25 minutes**

Servings: **4**

Ingredients:
- 5 quarts chicken broth
- 2 cups uncooked white rice
- 1 ½ cups celery, chopped
- 1 ½ cups red onion, chopped
- 1 tbsp. garlic, minced
- 8oz ground pork
- 8oz ground beef
- 2 tbsp. Cajun seasoning
- 1 tbsp. dried thyme

- 1 tbsp. dried parsley
- 1 tbsp. dried oregano

Directions :

1. Place the chicken stock, rice, celery, and 1 cup chopped onion in a large pot. Bring to a boil over high heat.
2. Reduce heat to medium-low, cover, and simmer until rice is tender, 20 to 25 minutes.
3. Meanwhile, place the remaining ½ cup of onion in a large skillet along with the garlic, pork and beef.
4. Cook and stir over medium-high heat until the meat is brown and crumbly.
5. Remove the excess fat, then add the meat to the cooked rice along with the thyme, parsley and oregano.
6. Mix well and serve.

Nutrition Facts: Calories: 134 Carbs: 27g Fat: 2g Protein: 4g

Tomato & Goat's Cheese Pizza

Preparation Time: **5 Minutes**

Cooking Time: **50 Minutes**

Servings: **2**

Ingredients:
- 8oz buckwheat flour
- 2 teaspoons dried yeast
- Pinch of salt
- 5fl oz. slightly water
- 1 tsp olive oil
- 3oz feta cheese, crumbled
- 3ozpassata or tomato paste
- 1 tomato, sliced
- 1 red onion, finely chopped
- 1oz rocket arugula leaves, chopped

Directions:
1. In a bowl combine all the ingredients for the pizza dough then let it rest for at least an hour until it has doubled in size.
2. Roll out the dough to the size you prefer.
3. Place the puree on the base and add the rest of the seasonings.
4. Bake at 400 ° F for 15-20 minutes or until golden at the edges and crisp and serve.

Nutrition Facts: Calories 387 kcal, Fat 9.9g, Carbohydrate 52g, Protein 8.4g

CPSIA information can be obtained
at www.ICGtesting.com
Printed in the USA
LVHW081631170621
690501LV00003B/44